Secrets To Curing Bad Breath

Michael L Dean

Disclaimer and Terms of Use: The contents of this book are not meant to substitute for any medical treatment, any visits or consultations with your health practitioner. Neither are the contents of this book meant to treat any health condition. The information herein is merely offered as an informational guide. As you read this book you should take no action for any health condition without the express knowledge and consent of your health-care practitioner. The information contained herein is purely for educational purposes only. None of it has been approved by the U.S. Food and Drug Administration. Your reliance upon information and content obtained by you at or through this publication is solely at your own risk. The author assumes no liability or responsibly for damage or injury to you, other persons, or property arising from any use of any product, information, idea, or instruction contained in the content provided to you through this book.

Contents

Introduction

No two individuals are alike. That means there is no one quite like you on the face of the planet anywhere. Sure, you may find your doppelganger hanging out in a café in Russia or your "twin" in downtown Peoria. But no one has the same chemical makeup that you have.

In fact, unless you have an identical twin out there you're the only one with the DNA you're carrying around with you right now. And even if you do have an identical twin, you are still quite unique in any number of ways. Just ask your closest friends and relatives.

This is a vital point to keep in mind while you read this book. You've probably noticed the title already, "Secrets to Curing Bad Breath" The key word here is "secrets". There is no single "secret" that miraculously fixes your breath while you sleep.

That's because of your glorious individuality. You are different from John Jones down the street who suffers from bad breath. Sorry John, no one told you that yet? Even if you both have bad breath that's caused by the same thing, the exact same remedies may not work on both of you.

Your chemical make-up, among other things is different. So as much as I wish I can say "take this and this" and – poof! – not a single person has bad breath any more, it just doesn't work like that.

As sad as it is, we've all come to expect a "one-size-fits-all" fix to health problems. That's because to a large extent the medical community, conspiring with the giant pharmaceutical companies have created that exact expectation within us.

Think about it. You walk into a doctor's office with high blood pressure. "Don't worry," your doctor says. "I've got just the thing to fix it."

And he whips out a prescription for a medication guaranteed to lower your blood pressure. You walk out of there happy that your physician has "solved" your problem.

One Size Does NOT Fit All

Even as you walk out of his office, your physician has already turned his attention to his next patient, who coincidentally has high blood pressure as well.

"Don't worry," he says again, "I've got just the thing to fix it." And he whips out a prescription for a medication guaranteed to lower this person's high blood pressure. Now, this individual is walking out of the office happy that his physician has "solved" his problem.

I think you're beginning to see a pattern here. In reality, your physician has not "fixed" your problem. He's merely masked it with some drugs.

He also did the exact same thing with the patient who came in after you with the same condition. When you stop using that drug, then you'll experience the return of the high blood pressure.

Medications, sorry to say, are not cures. Nor are they magic bullets that make you miraculously well. At best, they mask symptoms, such as pain, to help you "survive" your healing time a little more easily.

At worst, they cover up vital symptoms your body is using to tell you something isn't quite right. Sometimes we recognise this, sometimes we don't. We all have our moments and ways of dealing with this.

However, it does account for those expectations that every health problem has a single "cure" as it were and it just isn't so. The same treatment for halitosis, that's the medical term for this problem, doesn't work for everyone, even when the causes are the same.

It's just one of the given tenets that come along with natural remedies. That's why, you may have noticed, we've offered you a wide variety of possible solutions for your health problem.

The cause of your bad breath may differ widely from that of your brother's and this may mean a different approach and cure for you than it does for your brother.

Cookie cutter medicine, in which every one is treated as clones of each other, is not only wrong, but it's ineffective as well. Perhaps that's one of the reasons more individuals than ever before are turning to natural heath remedies.

Don't Become Impatient With Natural Remedies

Natural remedies may take a little longer to work. They, after all, work with your system.

They don't try to impose their timetable on your unique body. So, you may have to work your way through several of these natural remedy suggestions before you discover the one that works best for you.

You may think there's something wrong, as you try this remedy or that, you may get discouraged. Nothing works is what your conscious mind is saying. Why am I doing this? You may be asking only halfway through your search.

You're "doing this," I'll remind you, because you want to be rid of your bad breath. You may get impatient but if you continue your search, you'll discover that moment when you find the cure you knew was out there all the time.

Once you've discovered that, you've discovered one of the greatest joys of alternative and complimentary health!

You'll know it when you feel it, because it's a true healing, not just a cover up of the symptoms.

In this case, it's finally freedom from the bad breath which has been causing you untold misery.

It could be, in your particular case, that conventional medicine holds the key to an actual cure to your bad breath and that would be great too. You'd be way ahead of the game plan then.

In either case, you're now realising why one size therapy or treatment doesn't necessarily meet the needs of everyone including, possibly you.

The Best Way To Use This Book

You'll notice that I've included three different chapters dedicated solely to "cures." This doesn't mean that each and every one of these cures in each chapter is going to work for you but you do have a variety of ideas now.

Chapter 3 cures revolve around the remedies conventional medicine can provide you. If you try these or are already using these suggestions diligently and they don't or aren't working, don't fret. You're probably not doing anything wrong.

Your particular instance of less than fresh breath needs something different. That's all that means! That's where Chapter 4 comes into play. This chapter provides you some of the more common "cures" for bad breath.

These are cures your doctor may mention to you, but in all likelihood, you'd be set adrift on your own to find. Luckily, we've collected them here so you don't have to scour books . . . magazines . . . and hundreds of web sites searching for that one specific suggestion that works wonders on you. We've done the legwork for you!

Conventional Western Medical Therapy? Only One Source of Healing

Contrary to what many physicians, public health officials and others may want you to believe, conventional Western medical therapy may not be the most efficient system of healing when it comes to some health conditions.

Does this surprise you? Perhaps the fact that there are healing systems other than the conventional one we have in this country may. It's an eye-opener for many people when they discover other systems of healing.

Take for example, traditional Chinese medicine. Here's a good example of a system of medicine with a long, illustrious and frankly, quite successful history. But that didn't mean that Western doctors welcomed it in the country with open arms.

An Example : Acupuncture

One of the most effective forms of treatment that comes along with this system of medicine is acupuncture. It's proven itself over and over again to be an effective, drug free remedy for a host of various health conditions.

Surprisingly or maybe not so surprisingly, Western medical experts were slow to recognise the benefits of acupuncture and even slower to begin the adoption process of this wonderfully, wise system to help their patients.

We cover this particular remedy and more in the final chapter titled, appropriately enough "Homeopathy and More!" Like Traditional Chinese Medicine, Homeopathy is a healing modality and if you've never heard of it, we've spent a little bit of time detailing it here for you.

I realise that might be a bit out of the scope of the strict definitions of this book, but I do it for a very important reason. You're much more willing to try a remedy from this system, if you know a little about its background! If you already know something about homeopathy, great! If not, then you're in for a real eye opener!

Make This Book Work For You!

Dig into this book and read it through at least once. You'll no doubt recognise your symptoms, perhaps form some ideas on why you're experiencing bad breath and jump in and apply some of these remedies to your personal situation.

If none of these works and your bad breath continues, and you have yet to visit your dentist or physician, that might be your next step.

Perhaps your bad breath can't be treated with a simple cure. It may very well be that your situation has a more serious underlying health condition that needs to be corrected.

However you decide to use this book, I hope you find it useful!

CHAPTER 1:
BAD BREATH: AN OVERVIEW

In many ways, it's the ultimate personal problem. More than 50 million people suffer from chronic bad breath in this country. Fifty million. That's more than one third of the population.

You've probably tried to "fix" this problem yourself with various breath mints, sprays and mouthwashes. There are certainly enough of those products out there.

You've no doubt already noticed this. Stores are well stocked with mouthwashes. Check-out shelves are overflowing with breath mints of all flavors and brands. All in the hope that you don't have to enter the world with bad breath.

If you normally don't worry about your breath, you may, once you realise the number of products that are standing poised ready to correct it. Watch the television for any length of time. The commercials would have you believe there isn't a person alive who doesn't have this problem.

Well, in a strange sort of way that's true. Who among us hasn't experienced the coffee breath in the morning? Or onion breath after lunch? Or deadly morning breath when we wake up.

Have you ever tried not to treat yourself with some of these remedies when you suspect deep down in your heart, either the coffee or the onions or perhaps the garlic are lingering around a little longer than you think they should

But how many of us fight this problem day in and day out persistently, consistently?

Estimates have it that 50 to 80 million people in the US suffer from chronic halitosis.

That's probably more than any of us would have originally thought used these products like religious icons. That either tells us something about the power of advertising or our fear of social rejection!

Think about this: chronic, continued, persistent bad breath may be the result of a late stage liver disease. Then again, you can get bad breath as a result of developing a simple sinus infection.

The problem is that while you're experiencing your unpleasant breath, you really have little clue what the actual cause is. This is especially true when it comes to chronic bad breath. Short-term or acute bad breath can usually be detected with just a little common sense on your part.

What did you eat today right before you developed the problem? That single question usually takes care of the cause of the health condition.

Now, here's another statistic. About 90 percent of those who suffer with bad breath do so, **not as a side effect of some previously perceived problem.** At least that's what Dr. John Richter believes. He's a professional dentist practicing in the Philadelphia area.

The Complications Of Simple Bad Breath

As you might have guessed already, bad breath is not only a health problem, but a social problem as well. People with bad breath may be ostracised for reasons not entirely clear to them.

If you have bad breath, you may notice people step back from you when you talk or even as you're approaching them. You may notice that you don't quite hit that home run in the clubs like you used to with the opposite sex.

Or you do great on a date until it comes time to go home with him or her. You may even be adding these varied incidents up, but not quite able yet to connect all the dots.

It's one of those conditions few people tell you about. If you have less than fresh smelling breath, very few people feel comfortable mentioning it. And if you don't realise yet that you have it, you may be frustrated and confused.

How then do you discover you have it? You can't smell if your own breath odor is bad and none of your friends is ready to step up to the plate to tell you. Self diagnosis is just about impossible.

So the question lingers like a garlic smell in your mouth. If no one is willing to tell you and you have no easy way of knowing yourself, how do you tell if you have bad breath?

Some people claim it's impossible. But others, many dentists, dental experts and natural health providers included, have developed methods of self-testing.

Bad Breath: A Multi-Layer Problem

Bad breath is more than just a social problem. If the worst predicament you discovered about this health condition is that Liz isn't going to date you. Or Grant just won't kiss you, few doctors would be interested in studying the problem, let alone trying to find a solution.

No, those of you affected by less than sweet smelling breath are facing problems on a multitude of levels. Not the least of these is the professional level.

Having bad breath in the workplace can be highly uncomfortable at best. You may encounter less than pleasant greetings at meetings. This means not only you end up being self-conscious, but everyone you come in contact with does too.

And this is only the tip of the iceberg. Your bad breath just might be what's holding you from getting that much needed and very lucrative promotion. Try explaining that one the next time one of your creditors come knocking at your door. "I'd love to pay you what I owe you, but my bad breath is holding my promotion back and I just don't have the money to pay you right now!"

Less than good breath really is a social problem, even though I've already taken a flippant attitude toward it. If you do suffer from bad breath, then you know exactly what I mean. You're undoubtedly self conscious in all the usual social settings, from the cocktail party to the local barbecue to the meeting up with the group at the local pizza shop.

Before you know it, you'll feel uncomfortable and self-conscious enough that you'll simply refuse to do much of anything that involves other people.

On a personal level, bad breath can just about ruin your personal life. You'll end up avoiding discrete signs that your significant other would like to get a little more intimate. You'll pass on displays of affection.

You'll even begin to refuse to kiss your own children or your parents. You'll start, before too long, to feel totally isolated.

From Physiological To Psychological Problem

Simply put, bad breath can run the gamut of being a psychological as well as physiological problem. True, this condition starts out purely physiological. But it's hard to keep a condition like this out of the psychological realm of problems.

Actually, it's only a matter of time before you begin to exhibit some type of psychological issues in your daily affairs.

18

Looked at from one viewpoint, halitosis can be a larger psychological problem looming over your head than it is a physiological condition.

And because of this, you're undoubtedly feeling yourself avoiding certain situations now. Keep this up and before you know it, you may actually begin to lose contact with some of your very best friends.

So How Do You Tell If You Have Bad Breath?

Here are four very easy methods to discovering just this.

Lick the back of your hand. You may, by the way, want to do this when no one is looking! Allow a few seconds for it to dry. Then smell it. If it smells, you have what some refer to as a breath disorder.

Floss quickly a small area of your mouth. Smell the floss. Does it smell? If it does, you've got bad breath.

Here is a method that doesn't involve smelling. It just requires you to grab the tip of your tongue. Not an extremely easy task. Look in the mirror, grab the tip of your tongue, preferably with a washcloth.

Pull the tongue as far as you can. If you can see the very back of your tongue and it's whitish looking, this too may be a signal of bad breath.

Okay, so this next technique is really cheating in a way. It involves another person. But if you decide to use this one approach someone you trust and is quite gentle with words. Ask him or her, several times throughout the day, if your breath smells.

The Halimeter

Another way to determine if you have a breath disorder is to visit a dentist who has access to an instrument called a halimeter. This is an instrument that measures the concentration of certain chemicals in your mouth. Knowing this, your dentist can tell you the extent of your breath disorder, should you have one.

A Quick Look At The Cause

Recent research indicates that chemicals such as hydrogen sulfide, methyl mercaptan, as well as dimethyl sulfide contribute to bad breath. Collectively this group of chemicals is known as volatile sulfuric compounds. You may see them at times referred to by their abbreviation: VSC.

These chemicals are produced by anaerobic bacteria, which are found mostly on the back of the tongue.

They spend their lives "eating" or taking in nourishment, much like we do and then excreting the wastes. The waste products of these anaerobic bacteria are the VSC I've just mentioned.

Think about the smell of a rotten egg? Once you smell this distinctive odor you'll always recognise it. This specific and unique smell is caused by the sulfur compound hydrogen sulfide.

It really is the same smell that comes from feed lots as well as barnyards due to the sulfur compound methyl mercaptan.

Another sulfur smell comes from the ocean. This particular smell is due to the presence of dimethyl sulfide produced by Phytoplankton another microscopic lifeform.

Each of these various types of sulfur compounds, by the way, is also excreted as a waste product by the bacteria that like to live in our mouths.

When Is Volatile Not Quite Volatile?

These volatile sulfur compounds are not really volatile in the highly flammable or explosive sense as we know it. The term volatile when used as it is here means that the compounds have the capability of evaporating readily, even at normal temperatures and when they evaporate, they smell. When they smell, they offend. It's that simple.

If you're still recovering from the fact that bacteria produce waste products, wait till you hear this. They produce more than one kind of waste product. It's scary, but very true. And some of these other waste products have unique odors of their own. Here are just a few of them:

Various Waste Products Of Bacteria And Their Smells

Cadaverine. Did you notice the root word there? It is the smell that is normally encountered from a corpse. Another smell of bacteria in the mouth may be caused by the waste byproduct, putrescence.

It's the specific compound responsible for a large part of the foul breath odor associated with rotting and putrid meat.

But if you think that's all of the smells there is still one more that may be lurking within your mouth. This one is called **isovaleric acid.** I'm almost afraid to tell you what this odor resembles. Isovalaric acid can best be described as smelling like "sweaty feet."

Before you start strutting about thinking that you're exempt from these particular smells, be careful how you boast. No one, not one single one of us, is truly exempt from any of these smells.

In fact, your mouth alone is home for hundreds of different species of bacteria. Not only that, but you've got a battlefield raging in your mouth right now. Every single day, the bacteria are waging a serious battle between the types of bacteria. What is ultimately at stake in this battle between "good" and "evil?"

Nothing less than the quality and freshness of your breath. It's like a fully fledged motion picture plot being shot right inside your mouth, a cast of thousands, perhaps millions, and you don't even realise it.

The halimeter isn't the first instrument devised to test the severity or presence of bad breath.

But it does appear to be the most accurate one to date. It isn't in use everywhere yet and it's very likely that your dentist isn't using it. He may not even know that it's finally available.

If your dentist does use it, he won't use this in isolation though. Testing with the halimeter is merely part of an overall program, which includes, among other things, a thorough medical history, a physical examination as well as an emotional review of the individual too.

It's remarkable, actually. Dentists say that this instrument, within just a few short years, has been catapulted to the status of the premier instrument for the detection of chronic bad breath.

Before Any Type Of Treatment Begins

Before you expect some miracle cure for you bad breath, you and your doctor, if you're consulting one, need to then learn why the bad breath started in the first place. That's right! You need to know what is causing your malodor.

As we're about to see there are various reasons from incidental to quite serious for your bad breath. Once you know the cause, then you can begin your journey on curing it.

We've just learned that bacteria are the ultimate cause, but do you really know what attracts the bacteria and what increases their presence.

In the following chapter you'll ultimately learn about some foods to avoid, what foods to eat, what are bad habits and potential health problems.

So let's get on to the next chapter to discover some of these hidden reasons for bad breath.

CHAPTER 2:
CAUSES OF BAD BREATH

What we eat may very well affect the quality of our breath. And to a certain extent, we're all keenly aware of it. Think back to the last time you ate lunch and passed on the raw onions, because you had a one-on-one meeting with a very important client directly following your meal.

Onion breath was the last thing you needed and in all probability would not have made a stunning, professional impression.

We've all heard the remark on exactly why garlic is so effective at helping you stay healthy and free of colds. Your breath is so bad no one dare come within 25 feet of you and it's hard to catch a cold that way!

What You Eat Does Determine Your Breath

It's very true, your diet is probably one of the largest causes of bad breath. Exactly how that happens is interesting too. It's a touch more complicated than you might expect.

Once you eat, the food is eventually absorbed into the bloodstream. From there it's transferred into your lungs, where it's expelled. If you were like me, you thought the odors just lingered in your mouth. The odor won't dissipate until the body eventually eliminates the food.

Sure, in the meantime you can brush, floss and use mouthwash. That's one of those no brainers but this only masks the odor temporarily.

Not Brushing As A Cause

In fact, not brushing and not flossing may also be a cause of bad breath. In this case, the food particles really do linger in your mouth. While there, they attract bacteria.

Food particles love to hide between the teeth, on the tongue and around your gums. If not taken care of they can even begin to rot, leaving behind that lingering unpleasant smell.

In contrast, you may be surprised to learn, that those of you who diet regularly, may also develop bad breath and for the completely opposite reason: you don't eat often enough!

A related, but still different contributor to bad breath, especially the chronic type, is gum disease. Your dentist may call this periodontal disease. Plaque causes periodontal disease. It's a colorless, yet sticky film of bacteria that is constantly forming on your teeth. The bacteria create toxins which in turn irritate the gums.

In the more serious cases of gum disease, not only do the gums get damaged, but the bone and other structures supporting the teeth are damaged.

Got dry mouth? You might have bad breath too!

Xerostomia. You probably never heard of the word, unless you went to dental school. Xerostomia is what you and I call dry mouth. Dry mouth results when the usual, constant flow of saliva decreases for whatever reason.

This condition may be the result of any number of problems, including medications. Dry mouth may also result if you continually breathe through your mouth.

It's also a condition that increases the older you get. Now, don't go looking so smugly at the Baby Boomer sitting next to you. Your saliva begins to dry up the moment you reach your mid-20s!

Most cases of dry mouth begin, believe it or not, with prescription medication. The most notorious of these is those medications are prescribed to you due to high blood pressure or depression.

Before you say "that's not me," just read all the various medications and various medical conditions that can produce dry mouth. If you take any types of antihistamines, decongestants, or even painkillers you may experience dry mouth.

However that's not all. Here's a list of some of the other medications and medical conditions that are associated with dry mouth and perhaps your chronic bad breath:

1 Drugs for urinary incontinence
2 Drugs for Parkinson disease
3 Antidepressants

Realistically speaking, dry mouth is an adverse side effect of some 400 various medications! Yes, 400. Who would have ever thought! If you have any questions about whether one of the medications you're currently taking may be affecting the quality of breath, start your investigation with your prescribing physician or even the pharmacist.

If they can't give you a satisfactory answer, check out the medication on its official web site. If bad breath isn't listed as a side effect, don't give up. Find a number for the manufacturer of the medication you're taking and ask a customer service representative.

Why dry mouth Causes bad breath

Right about now, you're probably wondering what's the connection between dry mouth and bad breath. The drying action of the mouth irritates many of its soft tissues. Once irritated, they may become inflamed and more susceptible to infection.

One of the many important jobs of your saliva is to cleanse the area. Without the saliva present to do its job, bad breath as well as a host of other oral health problems can crop up.

Chronic Use Of Tobacco . . . In Any Form!

Do you use any type of tobacco products? Bad breath is frequently seen among those individuals who use tobacco in just about any form and tobacco may help promote gum disease.

Not only that, tobacco users are more likely to also suffer from periodontal disease and are at greater risk than non-tobacco users to develop periodontal disease.

So far the causes of bad breath are pretty straightforward and for the most part easily dealt with. But there are those instances where bad breath can be a symptom of another, more serious medical problem. Chronic problems with the quality of your breath may mean your body is warning you that a local infection is resting in the respiratory tract, your nose, throat, windpipe or even your lungs).

Or continued, chronic bad breath may be the result of sinusitis or a post nasal drip. But there have been instances where less than fresh breath has been the harbinger of chronic bronchitis, or diabetes.

Those who suffer from types of gastrointestinal disturbances may also experience persistent bad breath, as do people who have liver or kidney problems.

Specific Foods May Cause Bad Breath

We all know that garlic, onions and other sharp tasting foods can contribute to bad breath, at least temporarily. But, did you realise that there are a few more foods that may be hindering your fresh breath.

If you know this, then you can avoid eating these before you meet that special someone or go in for that big job interview or land that new client.

Milk and cheese, believe it or not, are two of the most offensive foods around and stop right there. It's not the fat content of the food that is giving you problems. So changing to low fat milk won't help you one bit.

If you are lactose intolerant, you may just not want to eat dairy products at all and this is regardless of whether you feel a physically adverse affect or not. This is difficult to do, I know.

The problem is that your body just can't digest these foods properly. So they are available to the bacteria in your system for a longer period of time.

Before you decide with certainty that you aren't lactose intolerant, read the results of this study, published in the Los Angeles Times, more than 10 years ago. It's a real eye-opener.

According to this research, nearly 67 percent of the American public is unable in some form to digest dairy products properly. Wow! That's a whopping two-thirds of us!

Now, think again! Are you sure you're not lactose intolerant?

Fish. Yes, fish can give you bad breath and we're just not talking about that fishy smell either. Because of the very high protein content in fish it can take a bad breath problem and exacerbate it.

Coffee Breath

This one you've probably seen coming: coffee. Yeah and don't think going decaffeinated helps. Coffee contains high levels of acids that cause the bacteria responsible for your bad breath to reproduce rapidly and create a bitter taste in your mouth. Keep the acidic content part of this sentence in mind. Any food high in acid content does the very same thing.

Want to stop your coffee breath today? here's a quick hint. Switch your drinking habits from coffee to tea. It's that easy. Okay, so it's easier said than done.

Think Alcohol!

We'll mention this again and again throughout this book but it's really important to realise that alcohol can cause bad breath. And it's more than just the fact that you drink it and the odor of the drink itself lingers with you.

Granted, that's bad enough. Alcohol itself is what's known as a "drying agent." In fact, it's one of the most commonly used drying agents in foods.

If you've used certain types of mouthwash, you may have noticed an alcohol content in it. You want to avoid this. It's only going to make your problem worse in the long run.

Chemically speaking, alcohol is a "desiccant", a drying agent. It's used in scientific laboratories to "dry out" hard to reach areas in test tubes and beakers.

When you put alcohol, in any form, in your mouth, you get the same result, a drying out process but don't think that if you don't use those mouthwashes, you're not killing bacteria.

The alcohol was never included for the purpose of killing them. The alcohol was included, now get this, so that the product looks nice on the shelf. Enough said!

What About Sugar?

Here's another place where sugar is the bad guy. Sugar just never seems to get a break. It's one of those foods we love, but has been proven time and time again, not that good for our overall system.

Avoiding sugar is extremely important if you have bad breath and stomach problems, especially flatulence. We've already talked about lactose intolerance and dairy products, if you recall. This warning of staying away from sugar is closely related to it.

Look at this way, sugar is just not good for your body in so many ways, this is just one more reason to try to keep your consumption of it as low as possible.

Instead of eating sugar, why not replace it with fresh fruits and vegetables. This works to help promote better breath in a couple of ways. First, it does eliminate the sugar flowing throughout your body and the bad breath, almost immediately.

But more than that, your body requires some time to digest fruits and vegetables. Eating more of these foods will help your system flush out toxins, like the bad bacteria that can eventually lead to the bad breath.

Bingo! You've just solved two sources of bad breath with one vital step of dietary change.

The next chapter talks about some of the cures for bad breath which your dentist may suggest when you visit him or her for this problem.

These are what I like to call "your more conventional" approaches to bad breath. They include small, simple changes you can make right now that will make a world of difference in the freshness of your breath.

CHAPTER 3:
CURES FOR BAD BREATH

It's not a bad idea you know. Oh, I know what you're considering. You're wondering if your breath is bad enough or chronic enough to visit a dentist.

Only you can make that decision but I can tell you, if you have decided to go, you can take a few steps to be prepared for it. Your dentist at the very least will ask you a few questions. And you can prepare yourself in a number of ways.

What you can do

For your part, don't eat, drink, chew gum or smoke three hours before your appointment and don't brush your teeth either for three hours before your visit.

If you're female, you can also make the visit go more smoothly if you don't wear any type of perfume, scented lotions or even a scented lipstick.

Any one of the products mentioned above may mask exactly what your dentist is looking for, a malodorous smell.

Taken any antibiotics within the last month? If you have then check with your dentist. Tell him you have. He may want to reschedule your appointment to a later date. These can also affect the state of your breath.

Once you get in to see your dentist, he will have some standard questions he'll ask you. I'm listing a few of them here. You might as well get started thinking about them now.

> When did the symptoms first appear or you first realised they were present?
> Do your symptoms appear only occasionally or are they chronic?
> How often do you brush your teeth?
> If you have dentures, how often do you clean your dentures?
> How often do you floss?
> What's your diet like? What types of food do you usually eat?
> Are you currently on any medications? If so, what kinds?
> Do you breathe through your mouth?
> Do you snore?
> Do you suffer from allergies or sinus problems?
> Do you have any ideas of what might be causing your bad breath?

➤ Have others noticed your breath?

Your dentist will probably then smell not only the breath that emanates from your mouth, but the breath from your nose as well. From here, he'll rate your odor. More than likely, he'll use a scale of zero to five. With zero being no odor and five, well, you get the picture.

Some dentists are now using the halimeter. We've talked quite a bit about it in an earlier chapter.

If there is no underlying medical problem, it's highly unlikely that your dentist will stray far from the standard advice of good dental hygiene.

He won't stray far either because for the majority of us, some portion or all of it works together quite nicely to help improve the quality of our breath.

The first of these is to brush your teeth after every meal. Yes, we've heard that from our mom over and over again. And yes, I do understand that in today's world, we eat more and more of our meals away from home.

But I do see people who take this advice to heart. They carry a toothbrush and toothpaste with them. Not a bad idea, actually and it's an especially good idea if you know that following a meal, your breath turns well, let's not use the term deadly.

There's no reason actually why you can't keep a toothbrush and some toothpaste stashed in your desk at work. At the very least, attempt to brush your teeth at least twice daily.

Floss once daily. And that's a minimum. You really should floss more often but if you can manage to floss at least once a day, you'll be doing good. If you've learned how to floss correctly, this one habit goes a long way to removing food particles and plaque from between your teeth.

Brush your tongue. Yes, you did read this one correctly. Brush your tongue. Now don't go scrubbing it down like it's the kitchen floor. But gently clean it. This single act removes dead cells, bacteria and food debris. In addition to gently brushing it, use a soft-bristle brush on your tongue.

Invest In A Tongue Scraper

You may also want to invest in a flexible tongue scraper. If you're not familiar with these, it's a device specifically designed to clean the tongue. Some scrapers have a loop in one end for you to be able to "scrub" the tongue to remove the germs and plaque.

There are several varieties on the market and they are relatively inexpensive. If you've invested in one and don't really like it, don't hesitate to try another style. The scraper does you absolutely no good if it just sits in your bathroom cabinet collecting dust.

Wear dentures? Keep 'em clean, too! Even if you only wear a partial or a bridge, you need to clean these just as thoroughly as you do your natural teeth. At the very least, you should clean your dentures once a day.

If you have any questions about your particular situation, don't hesitate to ask your dentist about how often you should be cleaning your false teeth.

Are Your False Teeth The Culprit

Here is a quick and easy way to see if your set is the cause of your bad breath. Remove your dentures. Place them in a sealed plastic bag, like one you'd store leftover food in. Obviously, you'll want to perform this experiment when you're not expecting any visitors.

Now seal the plastic bag. Allow it to sit without disturbing it for about five minutes. Crack the plastic bag open at the end of that period. Go ahead, you're ahead of me on this one I can tell, you're going to smell it.

Whatever you smell is pretty much what your breath smells like to others. Why, you may ask, do your dentures smell like that? Simple. Those bacteria that are lurking around, under and generally throughout your set of false teeth are causing that odor.

Let's face it, there's little difference between your false teeth and another person's "real" teeth. When you eat, no matter which type of teeth you have, you'll accumulate the same type of bacteria.

This cause for the malodorous breath is easily enough repaired. The solution is to diligently remove the offending bacteria as often as possible.

Many people don't give enough thought to cleaning their dentures. Many don't seem to clean them often enough. How often are you cleaning yours?

Let me explain why the cleaning of dentures is crucial in the restoration of healthy breath again. There's a space between your denture and your gum tissue. And this space is, imagine this! The natural location for bacterial growth!

Your Dentures Are Harboring Bacteria!

Bacteria call it home because, quite frankly, they feel pretty well protected here. But at the same time, microscopic food particles will also climb their way into this space. And these food particles, as you may already be surmising, provide a natural form of nourishment for the very alive bacteria.

So what should you do? In an ideal world, you should remove your dentures following every meal and clean them. You should brush your false teeth in this manner not only on the outside, but on the inside as well.

Do you use an adhesive to keep your teeth in place? Every time you take your dentures out to brush them, then you need to clean the old adhesive off and put some fresh on the teeth. And while you have your teeth off, very gently brush your gum tissue as well using only a soft-bristled toothbrush.

Now, having told you all of this, I also have to add that the material from which your dentures are made are pretty porous. This means they probably have a host of "nooks and crannies" where this halitosis causing bacteria can hide out for a while.

Keep in mind that the size of your toothbrushes bristles are no doubt giant in comparison to the size of these tiny holes in your denture. And this is where any number of bacteria may live.

Drink Water And Then More Water

Water. Water. And more water. It seems to be an answer to just about every health question these days. One of the reasons for this though is to keep your mouth moist.

And I'm not talking coffee here folks. I'm definitely not talking alcohol. And I don't mean increase your intake of soda or soft drinks. Water. Strictly water. Got it? Good.

Chew gum. Chewing gum naturally stimulates saliva and that helps to prevent your mouth from drying out, one of the major causes of bad breath.

Hold hard candy in your mouth. Preferably sugarless hard candy. This too will help create more saliva and in the long run keep your mouth from drying out.

Don't use an old toothbrush. You really should toss your old toothbrush every three to four months and buy a new one. Think about it. Bacteria collects on that brush.

And when you do buy your new brush, by the way, try to remember to get yourself a soft-bristled one.

Schedule and keep regular dental checkups. It's something we all dread unless I suppose you're the dentist doing the examination! But it's important for you to see a dentist twice a year, minimum. He'll not only examine your teeth during this appointment, but he may also clean them.

By all means don't argue with your dentist on this suggestion. Not only should you get your teeth cleaned, get as many of those cavities filled as possible as soon as possible. The bacteria that cause bad breath just love to hang out in cavities.

What about a Water Pik?

At one time, these things were under every Christmas tree in the United States. It's not a bad instrument to have. If you suffer from bad breath, be sure to use the water pik right after breakfast. And for extra protection, put an ounce of hydrogen peroxide in the water in this pik as well.

Another tip to practice is the simple "rinse-your-mouth-when-you're-away-from-home" trick. Plenty of us already do this now. For those of you who have never tried it, you should. Simply swish plain, ordinary water around your mouth and teeth following each snack or meal you eat. It really is that simple.

This, in effect reduces the food particles that linger as well as the drink residue, translate this into sugar, that can promote bad breath.

The remedies mentioned in this chapter all fall well within the realm of conventional Western medicine and common sense. In the next chapter, we explore some remedies that have been handed down from generation to generation.

While not all of these may be backed up by scientific evidence, the medical community is researching more folk and natural remedies than ever before and one of the most surprising things they're discovering is that they work!

So, if you found nothing that works or is relevant for you in this chapter, be patient. I've got another chapter lined up for you, chock full of more tips, tricks and techniques for curing bad breath.

CHAPTER 4:
NATURAL AND FOLK REMEDIES FOR BAD BREATH

Sometimes all you really need to do is look around your kitchen to discover a handful of proven remedies for bad breath. Hey, don't look so surprised. It's true! Humor me with this one!

Come on! Let's take a quick peek at your shelves right now. I'm confident we'll find something.

Look here, you've got apple cider vinegar. Here you go! Use apple cider vinegar as a mouthwash and you'll be using a bad breath cure. Dilute half a tablespoon of the liquid into a glass of water. Then gargle with it for a minimum of 10 seconds.

Didn't think we'd find a cure so soon, did you? Makes you wonder what else you have hiding in your kitchen cabinets.

Before you think you've found a miracle cure, let's look a little deeper at what this variety of vinegar really contains. It's long been known to be a natural bacteria-fighting agent. But more than that, it also contains a myriad of minerals and trace elements. Just look at some of them here:

potassium, calcium, magnesium phosphorous, sulfur, copper, iron silicon and fluorine.

Every one of those substances noted is needed in order to keep your body in a healthy state of balance.

Wait! Here's another bad breath cure in your kitchen cabinet. It's baking soda! Believe it or not, this is a fantastic remedy for less than clear breath and it does this by changing the pH balance or the acidity level in your mouth.

When you use baking soda, it makes your mouth less friendly as an environment for bacteria that ultimately causes bacteria. All you need to do is add some baking soda to your toothbrush, brush with it. Then simply rinse your mouth with water.

If you don't feel comfortable doing that, make a quick stop at your local grocery store or drug store. There are several brands of toothpaste that already have baking soda in there.

When you use this, though, remember to brush the top of your tongue. This helps to dislodge any particles contributing to your bad breath.

Look What We've Found In Your Refrigerator

We've already mentioned that sometimes bad breath is simply caused by dry mouth. Well, look what we've discovered in your fridge that can help this situation. Well, water of course. But, there are a few other things as well.

Sometimes eating a citrus fruit with its high citric acid content can help here. Your orange, lemon and grapefruit already here in the fridge can go a long way to improving your breath.

Specifically, the acid in the fruit stimulates your saliva production, which in turn helps to suppress some of the bacteria that cause the foul odor. But citrus works on another level. The tangy taste of the fruit helps to leave the mouth smelling fresh.

Here's another food that can help you in your quest to clean your breath. Try a cucumber. Yep. The lowly, unappreciated cucumber. This is an especially useful trick to use right after you've eaten lunch or supper.

Take a slice of this vegetable and press it up against the roof of your mouth. Hold there, if you can for about 30 seconds. This helps clear any bad breath loitering from your meal. It works due to the cucumber's phytochemical content. The specific phytochemicals in this vegetable kill the bacteria responsible for the odors. Pretty nifty, huh?

Fiber To The Rescue

Fiber has been touted as a cure for constipation, a godsend for those with diabetes, and up until several years ago, one of the best kept health secrets around. Would you believe that in addition to all its other attributes, fiber may also hold the key to improving your breath?

Fiber helps to remove the toxins that cause bad breath initially. At least according to Phyliss Balch, a widely known nutritionist and author of the book, *Prescription for Nutritional Healing.*

Oat bran, according to Balch is one of the best types of fiber for this purpose, but you can also use rice bran if you prefer. Another type of fiber she recommends to cure bad breath is psylium husks.

Psylium husk, if you've never heard of it, is the covering of the seeds of the Plantago Psylium plant, which is native to the Middle East. Most individuals use psylium to help improve digestion and indeed this is partly why it's recommended for bad breath. It'll help sweep the toxins out of your system quickly.

Be careful when you use this supplement, because it really is fiber rich. Some individuals, when they first begin using it, complain of bloating or of acquiring gas. Most health experts say when you start using this supplement, think small.

You should start off with small doses of the psylium for several weeks. Then carefully work up to a full, recommended dose of it.

I'd like to interject just one more word of warning it you're planning on using psylium to help improve the status of your breath. Some people discover that they are allergic to this supplement and we're not talking about just a few hives here and there sprinkled throughout your body.

Some who have used this, especially in larger quantities have experienced anaphylactic shock from the husk. This is the same reaction that many individuals experience when they are allergic to bee stings.

You'll recognise the symptoms of it almost immediately. And that might be the only good thing about it. You need to treat this condition immediately as well.

For the most part the major symptoms of anaphylactic shock include constriction of your airways, a light headedness and perhaps even fainting.

Other signs to watch out for include a swelling of the neck and face, as well as an itching and the development of low blood pressure.

Go Green, In Drinks, That Is!

It's a drink that has gained much popularity in the last several years. It's called a "green drink" in the most generic terms. But I'm sure with just a quick survey of your local health food store, you can probably find several different types and brands. No matter the brand or the specific make up of the drink, the main active component, natural health experts tell us, is chlorophyll.

Chlorophyll, the substance you normally associate with plants, actually is a thorough and effective cleansing agent when it comes to toxic build up in your body.

A quick zip through the internet or a short stroll through your local health food store proves quickly that there are many brands out there, all claiming to be the best!

The easiest way to use this type of product is to place a tablespoon of the powdered form in a glass of juice. Do this twice a day and you'll notice a difference.

If you prefer, you can use this supplement as a mouth rinse as well. Just take one tablespoon to a half a glass of water and rinse.

It might surprise you to learn that boosting certain vitamins and nutrients in your system helps to clear up bad breath. One of the first vitamins you may want to try is vitamin C.

When you get this at your local health food store, be sure that the product includes bioflavonoids. This combination works the best. This may seem like a large serving, but Balch recommends between 2,000 and 6,000 mg of vitamin C daily.

This vitamin is crucial in healing mouth and gum disease as well as preventing bleeding gums. But that's not all. This large serving of vitamin C also helps to rid your body of excessive amount of mucus as well as toxins which contribute to this condition.

Think Zinc!

So who says a pithy little saying that rhymes can't provide you with a useful health giving tool. Zinc, according to Balch, contains antibacterial properties, which makes it perfect to help improve your breath. But not only that, zinc also neutralizes sulfur compounds, a common cause of mouth odor.

When you think zinc and use zinc, don't use more than 100 mg a day. Your optimum serving is 30 mg three times a day.

Time to "restock" Your Good Bacteria

Perhaps your bad breath is telling you it's time to take a second look at the status of your body's "bacteria count." As you're probably well aware, your system needs a substantial amount of what known as "good bacteria" to keep your health balanced and your energy level vibrant.

What's not quite so widely known is that keeping your good bacteria count up helps to keep that bad breath at bay. If nothing else has worked to improve your condition, then perhaps you want to try this remedy.

Good bacteria, by the way, is called acidophilus and can be found at health food stores nationwide. If you can't find it at your local store, don't hesitate to get on the web to search. You can find many reputable sites selling it.

Really, You Want Me To Chew On Grape Seeds?

Please don't tell me the only way to get rid of chronic bad breath is to chew on grape seeds? That's what one of my friends told me. She read it on the web, she said!

No, thankfully, you don't have to chew on grape seeds to eliminate foul mouth odor. But, one remedy does involve grape seeds. But the grape seeds are taken as a supplement in a tablet or capsule form.

Still interested? If you are, read below to discover how this relatively new supplement, discovered within the last 20 years or so! can help cure the malodor in your mouth.

One of the trade names for this antioxidant is called pycnogenol, but if you can find a grape seed extract, you've discovered the supplement you may need to improve your bad breath.

Grape seed extract is a powerful free radical scavenger that acts as an anti-inflammatory. When you take this with vitamin C, you're enhancing the potency of the vitamin itself. Give it a try!

A vitamin you may want to check out is the B complex. Sometimes a deficiency of this family of nutrients can trigger bad breath. This is especially so with niacinimide. Try taking an extra 50 mg of this nutrient with each meal.

But don't let it stop there. You'll also want to take a high-potency B-complex tablet and perhaps even boost that with an extra B6, 50 mg once daily.

Herbal Remedies

Just as you can find any number of herbal remedies for a host of health problems, herbs can help cure your bad breath as well. You just need to know which herbs to use and how to use them.

One of the most widely used herbs is **Tea Tree Oil.** Many people for the last several hundred years and more have used this as a toothpaste "additive" All you need to do is add a drop of the oil into your toothpaste prior to brushing.

But if you're not satisfied with that, you can easily create a mouthwash from this oil. Take one cup of warm water and place three drops of tea tree oil in it. Gargle this up to three times a day, preferably right after you eat!

Keep in mind that you just gargle with this mixture, **never, ever** swallow it.

A variation of this rinse is to add peppermint and lemon oil to the tea tree oil. In fact, research has shown that the combination of these three essential oils was actually more effective than commercial mouthwash.

The results were measured by the level of volatile sulfur compounds that were left in the mouth following rinsing. As you'll recall from earlier in the book, many medical experts now believe an overwhelming number of cases of bad breath can be traced back to this single cause.

When you do eat, try munching on crunchy fruits and vegetables. You know the ones: apples, carrots, that sort of thing. These are the foods that can help remove food particles already stuck in your teeth as well as the bacteria and even help with plaque. Now you know why so many people call the apple "nature's toothbrush."

Carrying an apple or some carrots around in your purse or in your desk may be a great alternative if you just can't brush your teeth throughout the day.

If you've heard that alfalfa is a great cure for bad breath, you may be pleasantly surprised to learn how very easy it is to put this into action. All you simply have to do is take the tablet form of this herb. That's it.

If there's a part of you that doubts tablets could help, and you'd feel more comfortable with another method, think about the herb anise. According to herbalists, chewing anise, as well as fennel or cardamom seeds can also help control bad breath.

What? You've never heard of cardamom seeds? Neither had I until recently. It's a highly aromatic spice commonly used in the Eastern and Arab countries and believe it or not, even some Scandinavian countries.

It has a slightly sweet flavor. Its main use is for cooking, not for healing and shows up in a variety of dishes from fish to baked goods, even in some desserts.

If you're already familiar with this spice, you might already have it in your house.

And Speaking Of Fennel . . .

You can use fennel leaves in a number of ways. One of the easiest ways is to simply chew the leaves. This helps the saliva to start to collect in your mouth.

If you don't think you can handle chewing fennel leaves, it's alright. Herbalists say you can take the contents of a high-quality fennel capsule and mix it with another standby breath freshener, baking soda and brush your teeth.

Cloves, Anyone?

This herbal breath remedy is really no secret, though it's one we tend to forget about now and then. Let's talk cloves.

Cloves is a proven remedy for bad breath in that it has been used by a myriad of cultures worldwide for this very reason. One of the reasons for it popularity and it's effectiveness is that it's a potent antiseptic. You can benefit from this herb by merely taking three pieces of cloves, placing them in boiling water to use as a mouth wash.

Here's a remedy that appears totally oxymoronic. Bad breath can be helped by taking, are you ready for this? garlic supplements. Just doesn't seem right, now does it?

This may work though because garlic is a natural antibiotic. Taking it four times a day, two capsules a day, destroys the foreign bacteria in not only your mouth but your colon as well. Just a hint here and you may already be reaching for this type, you'll want to use the odorless form of garlic supplement. (Duh!)

Bees Use It Maybe You Should To

So what the heck is bee propolis and why is it good for your bad breath? Bee propolis has been a popular alternative health food supplement for decades now. It's known to provide your body with energy.

I'm betting you've never heard it as a remedy for bad breath. Propolis is a known antibacterial. Using this supplement helps to heal the gums, which we've already learnt contribute to bad breath.

Propolis by the way is the substance bees use to glue the materials of their hives together. They create this my mixing beeswax and other secretions with resins taken from the buds of conifer and poplar trees. These resins have natural germicidal properties.

If you plan on using this, just follow the directions on the label of the product.

Here are the ingredients of a mouthwash tea that is made expressly for combating bad breath. If nothing else seems to be working for you, why not try this?

You'll start by steeping two sprigs of coarsely chopped parsley, along with three whole cloves and a teaspoon of powdered myrrh in a pint of boiling water. Add to this one-quarter teaspoon of powdered goldenseal.

Stir this occasionally while its cooling. Then strain it. Don't drink it as a tea but instead use it as you would a mouthwash. This is also the perfect mouthwash for a sore throat.

Just when you think I couldn't come up with one more cure for bad breath, I still have a last chapter ready for you, whenever you are.

In the following chapter I talk about some of the other medical systems as well as cures for bad breath. Have you ever heard of homeopathy? It may hold out some hope that will help for your halitosis.

I also talk about Traditional Chinese Medicine as well as the medical system that comes to us from India, Ayurvedic medicine.

Are you ready to learn even more ways to make your breath fresh smelling? Once and for all. Keep on readin'!

Chapter 5:
HOMEOPATHIC AND MORE!

Conventional Western medicine isn't the only system of healing that effectively restores health. But that's not any great revelation. If you've ever used acupuncture to relieve any of your pain, you're already familiar with the traditional Chinese medicine.

While not associated with any one country, herbal medicine is a system of healing that has been widely promoted, used and celebrated world wide. Differences in herbal healing among countries is simply due to the types of plants found in various climates and countries. But the foundation of herbal medicine is the same, and has remained the same for literally thousands of years.

But homeopathy as a form of medicine? If you've never heard of it or its fundamental method of healing you may be a little skeptical at first.

I know I was. It did little to convince me of homeopathy's effectiveness to learn that England's royal family had used it for years and years.

I was curious though. I soon learned that homeopathy is a system of medicine based on the theory that you treat the individual's health condition by administering a highly diluted substance.

This substance then triggers the body's natural system of healing. What substances you used to treat a person depended on the symptoms of the health condition itself, much as western medicine does.

The fundamental tenet of homeopathy is what we may consider the unlikely concept of "like cures like." In essence, this means that the substance that is the cause of the symptoms is used to cure those same symptoms in an illness.

A perfect example of this is when a person is administered cofea for insomnia. Cofea is a remedy made from coffee not your typical cure for the inability to sleep!

Of course, it didn't help me at all to learn that science has yet to explain homeopathy's effectiveness. And yes, despite your skepticism, it is very effective for some individuals for some conditions.

However, I'm now learning that some of the knowledge gained in quantum physics helps to explain some of the reasons why homeopathic medicine does work and it may even help me if I knew something about quantum physics.

Homeopathy must have something going for it, though, I began to realise. After all, it has been used worldwide for more than two centuries.

But more than that, its theories have been used for even longer. The theories were developed and practiced as far back as ancient Greece.

Hahneman Organised Homeopathy As a System

It was not until Samuel Hahneman, who in 1796 actually developed both the scientific and the philosophical underpinnings of this treatment that it become an organised form of healing. His brilliance drew all the knowledge together to create a usable and methodical system of medicine.

What really excites many of us who now use it though is that it can be implemented right along with just about any conventional medical treatment.

If you haven't guessed yet, homeopathic remedies are unique energy medicines, drawn not only from the plant world like herbal medicine, but also the mineral and animal worlds.

I mentioned earlier that all of the medicines used are highly diluted before they are used. In fact, some of the "cures" are so highly diluted that not even an entire molecule is left intact.

The key to their effectiveness is that they are said to gently boost the natural energy of the body. The substances used are extremely safe, even for pregnant women and those who are very sensitive.

Traditional Chinese Medicine

Then there's the system of medicine known as Chinese medicine. The Chinese bring to this country a vastly different view of looking at medicine and an intriguing new way of treatment.

That includes the practice of acupuncture for bad breath. Yes, indeed, believe it or not, acupuncture may actually help your bad breath odor.

To truly understand what's happening, though, we have to learn just a little bit about what's known in this country as Traditional Chinese Medicine. You may see this abbreviated in books or magazines simple as TCM.

This system of medicine asserts that bad breath may be caused by the digestive system that isn't functioning properly. Many experts in the Chinese Tradition blame the stomach heat which is emanating from this organ.

This "heat" could mean in the language of the Chinese medical community that you're eating an improper diet, not getting enough rest or even experiencing a prolonged illness. Or, it could be Chinese traditionalists suggest, the results of an excessive amount of stress.

When you discover an experienced and licensed acupuncturist, he or she can identify whether you have this "internal heat" simply by taking your pulse. Difficult to believe, perhaps, but . . .

Once this "heat" is determined to be present, then the acupuncturist will have you undergo the treatment. The purpose is to "balance" your system and "harmonise the "yin and yang" of your body.

Acupuncture

If you're not familiar with the nuts and bolts of acupuncture, you may be interested in learning that the treatment involves the placement of very thin needles in various areas of your body.

These needles are lined up with certain, predetermined meridians of your body which throughout the thousands of years acupuncture has been used, have proven to be the most beneficial for the ailment from which you're suffering.

Traditional Chinese medicine also recognises that bad breath may be helped by eating what is known in that medical system as bitter food. These include Belgian endive and other dark green, leafy vegetables.

This system of medicine also advises against drinking large amounts of coffee, alcohol, sugar milk as well as fried and spicy foods. Practitioners of Chinese medicine agree with the Western experts that these foods contribute to the problem.

But it also promotes the consumption of water. In fact, like Western medicine, traditional Chinese medicinal healers advocate that their patients drink plenty of fluids and the reason goes beyond the simple Western explanation of "keeping the mouth moist."

Again, in this system of health, the reason once again harkens back to the amount of "heat" you may have in your stomach at any one time. Water, as well as soup help to restore balance to your system. This in turn reduces heat in your stomach.

If you're like many people, you may find it difficult to drink enough water throughout the day. If that's the case, why not try to eat more fruits and vegetables. These foods contain various juices that can act like and in some cases actually be converted into water.

The Ayurvedic Method

The oldest existing medical system, ayurvedic originated in India some 4,000 years ago, that's some 2,000 years before the birth of Christ!

It's a well rounded and well proven method of healing that encompasses more than just a listing of herbs and how to use them for your specific health ailments. Far from it, the amazing aspect of this ancient medical approach is how intricate it really is.

Yes, Ayurvedic medicine does use herbs to help heal your body, but it also utilises other natural therapies as well as an astonishingly well developed diet.

In all of this, Ayurvedic declares that treatment just isn't tailored to you, but to your body type as described by this medical system, which places equal emphasis on the body, mind and spirit.

The bottom line of Ayurvedic medicine is its attempt to restore the natural harmony of your body.

Ayurvedic isn't a word that flows off our tongue very easily. Actually, it's a Sanskrit word meaning "the science of lifespan." Technically, the word comes from two distinct parts. The first part of the word, "ayur" means life. And the second portion of the word, "veda" means knowledge.

According to ayurvedic medicine, the human body is made of five basic elements: space, air, water, fire and earth. The human being, according to this ancient medical system, is nothing more and nothing less than a miniature of nature.

Having said that though, this system of medicine recognises three distinct body types called doshas by many. These three doshas explain not only the actions and gestures of you as an individual, but the doshas also help to explain the activity of your individual metabolism in many cases.

If your immediate thought of Ayurvedic medicine is in the form of the doctor and author Deepak Chopra, MD, I'm not surprised. While he is a Western-trained endocrinologist, he is also one of the most outspoken advocates for Ayurvedic medicine.

You'll notice that Ayurvedic medicine, even in attempting to find a cure for bad breath, cares far more deeply about what is actually causing the problems at times than Western medicine appears to be.

You'll have a host of different herbs and treatments for bad breath depending on what the Ayurvedic doctor has determined to be the initial cause of the malodor.

Ama

Haven't heard of that word? Not surprising. That's the word Ayurvedic medicine uses to describe that thick coating on the tongue. According to ayurveda, it could indicate more than just an unpleasant appearance. It may very well be a harbinger of bad breath.

Ama is though to be caused by an incomplete or an improper digestive process and it's also seen as the cause of bad breath.

In this area, Ayurveda and Western medicine are in complete agreement. Scrape the tongue clean and eliminate the bad breath. Even better though is to improve your digestive process!

Don't have a scraper available to you? Then your toothbrush works just fine. Remember though not to "scrape" too hard. Brush your tongue gently. After you've brushed, rinse your mouth thoroughly.

If the problem is merely that daily dental hygiene is not being followed, then this ancient system of therapy offers a wide range of "medicines" which can be used regularly between dental brushings. The first step is to take the astringent herb, Bakul, already a known aid in dental problems and rinse your mouth in a water solution that contains this specific herb at least twice daily.

Not only will you notice that your breath is consistently fresher, but that your teeth are being strengthened in the process. Bakul also has the reputation in Ayurvedic medicine as helping to keep the gums healthy.

Ayurvedic medicine also says that chewing on cumin can help rid you of bad breath.

In addition, this system of treatment offers a wide range of alternatives from Kapur, whose scientific name is cinnamon camphora, which helps treat the gum disease which is promoting the odor. Other similar herbs and "medicines" include but are in no way limited to Lavang, Supari, Sphatik, Mayaphal, and Elaichi.

Additionally, several other Ayurvedic therapies may also work. These are Jeerak, Manijishtha as well as Marich, and Kulinjan.

Every medicine mentioned here may be taken in one or more of three ways. Each is available as a powder so you can mix with water and rinse your mouth. All of these can also be found as both a tooth paste and a mouth wash.

If your bad breath is caused by a more serious underlying problem, then other medicines are usually recommended. Halitosis caused by a respiratory tract infection can be treated with medicines like Sitopaladi-Chuma, Talisadi-Chuma as well as Shrung-Bhasma.

A Gastrointestinal Infection

Another possible cause of your bad breath, according to Ayurvedic doctors is an infection originating in the gastrointestinal tract. And yes, this type of bad breath needs yet a different type of medicine in order to be dealt with effectively.

Many of the doctors use Triphala, three fruits as well as Trikatu, three pungent herbs. They may also tell their patients to take Kataj or Laghu-Sutshekhar.

Triphala, for example, can be found on line and in many local health shops in supplement form. It's described as a supplement that not only restores the natural balance to your body but also detoxifies and rejuvenates your system as well.

In additional to naturally cleansing your system, Triphala, gently maintains regularity while nourishing and rejuvenating your tissues. But that's not all, this specific medicine also helps to support healthy digestion and absorption.

Similarly, Trikatu promotes healthy digestion as well as absorption. Its name is derived from its composition. Trikatu literally means "three pungents." It is composed of ginger, black pepper and the lesser-known herb pippali.

A powerful healing formula, this specific medicine is said to support a healthy metabolism as well as help the digestion of your system. This particular medicine is also recommended by Ayurvedic specialists for those who want to lose weight.

Now if you're left, right about now scratching your head about these various natural remedies, I really don't blame you. Many of the names of these herbal medicines aren't familiar to us.

They don't roll off the tongue like chamomile or hawthorn do. That doesn't mean though that Ayurvedic medicine can't be a powerful, natural force in your natural health program. And it very well could be that you want to start right now.

But I urge you if you think that you might be even a little interested in Ayurvedic medicine, to do more research on it. For one thing, it's fascinating.

But in this way, you'll also discover whether it's a road you want to travel. Check it out not only on line, but with others in your area. Your local health food stores will probably know the name and location of an Ayurvedic practitioner.

You may be surprised too if you happen to mention it to your relatives and friends. You may discover they already know of individuals working with the Eastern form of medicine.

Yoga And Your (Bad) Breath

One of the fundamental causes of bad breath according to just about every system of medicine including conventional Western medicine is stress. Doesn't it seem as if stress affects absolutely every level of our health?

Just read the results of this one recent study. It examined in young men who practiced good oral hygiene and were in general good health. The study discovered that as their levels of stress increased, so did the production of volatile sulfur compounds in the mouth. In essence, as they got more stressed, their breath became less fresh.

The ultimate solution? Learn how to intelligently manage your stress. There are many ways of doing this, not the least of which is... you guessed it yoga.

If you've never taken a yoga course before, or bought a book on it and practiced it, you're in for a real treat. Not only will this system of exercise actually relieve your stress, but it will improve the health of just about every part of your body.

In addition to your stress being lifted from your muscles and bones and yes even your mind you'll discover that you'll have more energy and a renewed outlook on life.

Conclusion

Some people may see it as a nuisance a small blip on the radar screen of life. But for others, especially if the underlying cause of this irritating health condition is a serious infection, it could spell big problems for your health.

How you view bad breath depends on what happens to be the underlying cause. For the vast majority of us it's not a problem that leads to anything more serious. But for some it certainly is.

I hope that if you've taken anything away with you from this book, it's knowing that the cause of your bad breath may be total different from John Jones down the road.

And Mary in the next cubicle at work has a totally different cause for hers than either you or John!

That means, more than any other condition around, the remedies for bad breath will be just as individualised. How you ended up using this book, depended, of course, largely on the ultimate cause of your bad breath. From mild "garlicky" breath to halitosis caused by a more severe health condition, your treatment was tailored just for you.

I'm so glad you've eliminated your bad breath. I'm also pleased and quite honored that some suggestion or remedy you found in this book was able to help you.

Keep this book handy. You may have need someday of using it again if not for yourself, maybe for a family member or a friend. Hopefully, it'll be just as useful the second time around as it was this time.